HOW AN EXPERIENCED TCM DOCTOR TREATS BOWEL CANCER

First edition. February 3, 2024.

Copyright © 2024 yingxiong feng.

ISBN: 979-8224302413

Written by yingxiong feng.

How An Experienced TCM Doctor Treats Bowel Cancer

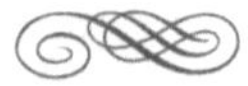

Yingxiong Feng

Introduction

Bowel cancer remains a significant health concern in the United States. It is one of the most common cancers diagnosed and a leading cause of cancer-related deaths.

The risk of bowel cancer increases with age, and a significant percentage of cases occur in individuals aged 50 and older.

Chinese Internal Medicine offers an alternative that elucidates the etiology, pathogenesis, syndrome characteristics, and principles of differentiation and treatment, as well as the rules for prevention, recovery, and regulation of internal diseases based on TCM theory.

The author's clinical experience and his journey to curing ulcerative colitis serve as a guidance for patients looking for better solutions for cancer treatment related to the colon and the bowel.

About The Author:

The author is a TCM doctor, teacher and Buddhist practitioner. He has published 20 books in Buddhism, culture and health.

Praised by many as "The best TCM doctor in New York Chinatown", "Loved by all his patients", "Patients' last hope".

Chapter 1

Ulcerative Colitis May Lead To Bowel Cancer

I start with my own story.

I migrated to Australia in 2003. Initially, I thought that with Australia's good water, clean air, and rich, healthy food, I could be more relaxed about my diet, following local customs. So, in the first two years, I often visited McDonald and KFC and ate other grilled and fried foods. Some days in 2006, I found irregularities in the toilets and was later diagnosed with ulcerative colitis. Going to the toilet and finding blood in my stool was very troublesome and unsettling.

I spent a week in Sydney's St. George Hospital and underwent routine colon screening, examination, and treatment by doctors. For most of the following two months, I had to insert some paste-like substance (not a suppository) into my rectum every day. Although this process was somewhat helpful, it did not solve the problem.

I had studied Traditional Chinese Medicine (TCM) before and had a general idea of how diseases occur and develop. I could then cop with some minor health problems with my basic knowledge of TCM. This was the first time I saw the problem too serious and was out of my own control.

I went to Foshan Hospital in China for another colonoscopy. Taking the advice of a Chinese physician, I began a combination of Western and traditional Chinese medicine, including herbal treatments for hemorrhoids. When I had my spare time, I looked deeper into TCM by researching books, trying to find a better solution to my problem.

After returning to Sydney, in addition to taking Chinese herbal medicine regularly, I also started to try making my own formulations. I realized that one of the main factors of my disease was my lifestyle and the foods I ate. As I was practicing Buddhism, over the next ten years, I completely changed my eating habits and became a vegetarian.

In about six months, my problem was solved, and the ulcerative colitis "disappeared." In about ten years, I was very careful about foods I ate. However, ten years later, the same problem occurred again, with blood in my stools and increased frequency of toilet visits.

I was hospitalized again at St. George Hospital. I thought that after ten years, there might be new drugs or better treatments available in Australia. Unfortunately, the doctors told me the same story and asked me to undergo the same treatment process.

I refused the medical advice of the hospital. I told the doctors: "I want to be discharged immediately and try to treat this disease myself." The hospital required me to sign a letter to waive their responsibility, allowing me to leave without undergoing treatment.

I tried the same Chinese medicine approach and improved my own herbal formulas. This time, the situation became easier, and I returned to normal in about two months. However, the problem was not fundamentally solved. Two years later, my intestines bled for the third time. This time it became more and more serious. In addition to ulcerative colitis, I also had internal hemorrhoids and anal fissures. My regular treatments were not effective, and the problem persisted for five to six months. For a while, sometimes it was better, but other times it was not. I had to delve deeper into clinical treatments of colon cancers and conduct more research into Huangdi Neijing (The Yellow Emperor's Inner Canon) and other TCM classics.

One of the factors I explored for the recurrence of the illness was that my decade of vegetarianism had gone to an extreme, making my constitution too 'cold.' Huang Yuanyu, a representative of the Yang-supporting school and physician to Emperor Qianlong, said, "Pure

Yang leads to immortality, pure Yin to ghosts. Excess Yang brings strength, excess Yin brings illness. Illness from Yin deficiency is one in a thousand; illness from Yang deficiency is in everyone. Later generations of medical practice have deviated, opening the door to nourishing Yin, indiscriminately treating people with Yang deficiency with Yin-nourishing medicine, a mistake that has persisted through the ages, truly deplorable." Life experience made me realize that our thoughts change with the environment and understanding. One must not rigidly cling to a fixed idea and must not follow a path blindly to its extreme.

Common symptoms of colitis include abdominal pain, increased bowel sounds, bloody stools, diarrhea, fever, rectal pain, weight loss, and malnutrition. My symptoms were not so severe as to include all these signs.

Tens of thousands of Australians suffer from ulcerative colitis and even colorectal cancer. Statistics show that about six thousand people are added to this list every year. Generally, doctors may prescribe various medications, most of which also have side effects. If the patient encounters very serious problems, surgery is necessary.

According to my doctor: Currently, there are no non-surgical treatments for UC. The treatment of this disease is only aimed at prolonging remission periods and reducing the severity of outbreaks.

This type of colitis is certainly one of the most difficult diseases to cure. Because each of us must eat and use the toilet every day. Using the toilet can affect the recovery process and often worsens the problem. But we must eat, and during recovery, we need food to keep us healthy.

Apart from surgery, there are several medications available in Australia for the treatment of ulcerative colitis. For example, sulfasalazine, which can have side effects such as headaches, nausea, diarrhea, and abdominal pain. For acute attacks or relapses, corticosteroids can be used to reduce inflammation, but these drugs can cause mood changes, osteoporosis, and diabetes. There are also immunosuppressive drugs like azathioprine, which can easily damage the liver and increase the risk of cancer.

Additionally, the Australian-made Predsol suppository helps with the inflammation of the disease. After trying 30 suppositories, it did not work for me. Rectogesic ointment, bought from a local pharmacy for hemorrhoids, has side effects (can harm the heart). I also used Proctosedyl ointment and Anusol suppositories, with unsatisfactory results.

I attempted to research more authoritative treatment plans in the Australian medical community, but the results were disappointing. The deeper I delved, the more I realized the superficiality and simplicity of Western medicine. Beyond the physical aspect, Western medicine's understanding of the true nature of life is almost non-existent. Not to mention their ignorance of meridian points and the relationship between yin-yang, the five elements, and the five zang-organs and six fu-organs; they don't even know why most patients with colitis and diarrhea should not drink milk.

My problem was also accompanied by hemorrhoids. I used Jiuhuashan Musk Hemorrhoid Ointment and Ma Ying Long's traditional Chinese medicine formula, but the results were also unsatisfactory. However, I am convinced that traditional Chinese medicine has better experience and methods. To study this disease and cure my problem, I consulted several traditional Chinese medicine practitioners and took the herbal medicine they prescribed. Sometimes, their medicine made my condition worse, and my bleeding became more severe. Although I knew that some of their formulas were not ideal, I still took the medicine, just to experiment on myself and make it a part of my practice of traditional Chinese medicine.

The proverb goes: "Illness enters through the mouth." Among various factors, an unhealthy diet is the main cause of my suffering from ulcerative colitis. Managing the stomach and ensuring its normal digestion is a key factor. The recurrence during the treatment process is closely related to personal emotions. In traditional Chinese medicine, such diseases often fall under the category of Yangming syndrome. Even in the case of colorectal cancer, it is frequently associated with both Yangming and Taiyin syndromes. Traditional Chinese medicine holds the belief that "Yangming syndrome does not lead to death," so theoretically speaking, colorectal cancer is easier to treat than other types of cancer. Patients should build confidence and not be afraid.

Over the past ten years, I have conducted in-depth research on this disease and tried dozens of herbal formulas targeted at my problem, finding effective methods.

Today, I can say that I have found a relatively ideal final solution. I think the symptoms of colorectal cancer should also be treated in this way. My solution involves three steps: First, harmonization to harmonize Shaoyang; second, purgation to clear damp-heat and intestinal toxins; third, tonification to nourish and support the righteous qi. During this, one should adapt to the specific conditions of deficiency and excess, cold and heat. Additionally, attention should be paid to daily diet, avoiding spicy, raw, and hard fruits, among others.

I cannot yet claim complete mastery, but on the path to understanding, my confidence has only grown stronger.

The "Huangdi Neijing" states: "Blood and qi are fond of warmth and averse to cold. When cold, they stagnate and do not flow; when warm, they disperse and leave." These few words are essential for treating blood disorders.

By treating my intestinal blood disorder, other issues related to the heart, liver, lungs, etc., were also resolved, and my sleep returned to normal, improving my overall ecological environment. I believe this is something that Western medicine absolutely struggles to achieve.

Chapter 2

Lifestyle And Eating Habits Are Main Factors OF Bowel Cancer

You are what you eat

Bowel cancer remains a significant health concern in the United States. It is one of the most common cancers diagnosed and a leading cause of cancer-related deaths.

Bowel cancer, also known as colorectal cancer, is a prevalent and potentially deadly disease that affects the colon or rectum. While genetics plays a role in predisposition, there is mounting evidence that lifestyle and eating habits significantly contribute to the development of bowel cancer. Understanding these factors is crucial for adopting preventive measures and promoting a healthier, cancer-resistant lifestyle.

Many Americans consume a diet rich in processed foods, which are often high in unhealthy fats, sugars, and sodium. These foods include packaged snacks, sugary beverages, fast food, and ready-to-eat meals. Excessive intake of these foods can lead to weight gain, inflammation, and chronic diseases.

The saying "you are what you eat" holds profound truth when it comes to bowel cancer. Diets rich in processed foods, red and processed meats, and low in fiber have been linked to an increased risk of colorectal cancer. High consumption of red and processed meats introduces harmful substances, such as heme iron and nitrites, into the digestive system, potentially leading to the formation of cancerous cells.

Portion sizes in the U.S. are significantly larger than those recommended for a healthy diet. Large portions at restaurants and the habit of consuming large quantities of food contribute to overeating and weight gain.

Conversely, diets abundant in fruits, vegetables, and whole grains provide essential nutrients and fiber that promote a healthy digestive system. Fiber aids in maintaining regular bowel movements, preventing the accumulation of carcinogenic substances in the colon.

Despite the known health benefits of fruits and vegetables, many Americans do not consume enough of these nutrient-rich foods.

Sedentary lifestyles have become increasingly common in modern society, and this lack of physical activity is another factor contributing to bowel cancer. Regular exercise not only helps maintain a healthy body weight but also promotes proper bowel function. Physical activity has been shown to reduce inflammation and improve the overall health of the digestive system, lowering the risk of colorectal cancer.

A sedentary lifestyle is prevalent in the United States, with many individuals spending excessive amounts of time sitting, whether for work, commuting, or leisure activities like watching TV. Physical inactivity is a significant risk factor for numerous health conditions, including cardiovascular diseases and obesity.

Being overweight or obese is a well-established risk factor for various cancers, including bowel cancer. Excess body fat, especially around the abdomen, can lead to chronic inflammation and insulin resistance, creating an environment conducive to the development of cancer cells. Maintaining a healthy weight through balanced nutrition and regular exercise is crucial in reducing the risk of bowel cancer.

High intake of sugary beverages, such as sodas and fruit-flavored drinks, along with snacks high in sugar, contributes to obesity, type 2 diabetes, and dental problems. These items are staples in many Americans' diets.

Eating out frequently at restaurants, especially fast-food establishments, can lead to unhealthy eating habits due to the tendency of these meals to be higher in calories, fat, and sodium than home-cooked meals.

Tobacco smoking and excessive alcohol consumption have been linked to an increased risk of colorectal cancer. Both substances introduce harmful chemicals into the body, promoting inflammation and damaging the DNA in the cells lining the colon and rectum. Quitting smoking and moderating alcohol intake are essential steps in reducing the risk of developing bowel cancer.

Many Americans do not meet the recommended levels of physical activity, contributing to the obesity epidemic and related health problems. Regular physical activity is crucial for maintaining a healthy weight and preventing chronic diseases.

According to the American Cancer Society, colorectal cancer is expected to affect a considerable number of individuals each year.

The risk of bowel cancer increases with age, and a significant percentage of cases occur in individuals aged 50 and older.

More about eating habits and lifestyle

THERE ARE SIGNIFICANT differences in dietary habits between Eastern and Western cultures, reflecting distinct understandings of food, eating practices, and the values associated with them.

Eastern diets, represented by China, Japan, and Korea, emphasize the balance and harmony of food. They typically include staples like rice, noodles, vegetables, and tofu, along with moderate amounts of fish and meat. Cooking methods focus on preserving the natural flavors of ingredients, emphasizing a light and nutritious approach.

Eastern cuisine underscores the balance and harmony of ingredients, with staples such as rice, noodles, legumes, vegetables, and seafood. Fish, seafood, and tofu are widely used, emphasizing a light and natural taste.

Eastern cooking prioritizes the authentic flavors of ingredients, employing methods like steaming, stir-frying, stewing, and boiling to maintain freshness and nutritional value. Eastern kitchens often use seasonings like soy sauce, ginger, garlic, five-spice powder, and Sichuan peppercorns to enhance the natural taste of ingredients.

In contrast, Western diets place a greater emphasis on meat, particularly beef, pork, and poultry, often accompanied by staples like bread and potatoes. Western cooking methods often emphasize frying and grilling, aiming for robust flavors in food.

Western cuisine heavily incorporates dairy products, bread, and potatoes as staples. It typically seeks strong flavors through methods such as baking, frying, and stewing.

Western cooking prioritizes the use of various herbs, butter, cheese, vinegar, and other ingredients to enrich and intensify the taste of food.

Compared to Eastern cultures, Western diets involve a higher consumption of dairy, with milk being a common component. While moderate milk intake is beneficial for health, concerns may arise regarding the feed used in modern dairy farming, as it may contain substances that could potentially be harmful to human health.

For example, some cattle feed may include antibiotics to prevent or treat diseases, enhancing the productivity of the cattle. However, prolonged consumption of dairy products containing antibiotics could lead to antibiotic resistance issues.

Growth hormones and hormone promoters are sometimes used to stimulate the growth and milk production of cows. Despite the existence of regulations in many countries to ensure the safety of hormone levels in dairy products, concerns persist regarding the potential impact of hormone residues on human health.

Some cows may be fed with genetically modified feed, and the consumption of such components by humans may have adverse consequences.

If the feed consumed by cows is contaminated with pesticides, these pesticides may potentially remain in dairy products, posing potential health risks to humans.

Additionally, certain regions may have heavy metals present in the soil and water sources. If these heavy metals find their way into the feed given to cows, it could result in an elevated presence of heavy metals in dairy products, posing a potential threat to human health.

Common belief holds that moderate milk consumption is generally beneficial for bone health since milk is a rich source of calcium, crucial for the development and maintenance of bones. However, some studies suggest a link between high calcium intake and an increased risk of fractures. This may be attributed to an excess of calcium leading to an imbalance of other minerals in the body, impacting the structure and strength of bones.

Excessive absorption of calcium from overconsumption of milk can potentially have adverse effects on the heart, kidneys, and other organs. Relying excessively on milk as the primary source of calcium may result in deficiencies of other essential nutrients.

Some individuals may experience lactose intolerance, making it challenging for them to digest lactose in milk. Others may have a milk protein allergy, leading to allergic symptoms such as shortness of breath and hives.

Now, let's discuss lifestyle changes. Currently, both in the East and the West, outdoor barbecue is a popular social activity, but prolonged and excessive consumption may be associated with some health issues.

During the barbecue process, the interaction between meat, fish, or other protein-rich foods and the heat source in the grill can generate carcinogenic substances such as polycyclic aromatic hydrocarbons (PAHs) and heterocyclic amines (HCAs). These substances are believed to be linked to an increased risk of cancer.

The smoke and caramelization products produced during barbecue may be detrimental to health. The interaction of caramelization products with sugar and protein can lead to the formation of harmful compounds.

Many barbecue foods are often rich in fat and calories, especially processed and marinated meats, sausages, and the like. Excessive consumption of high-fat, high-calorie foods may lead to weight gain, cardiovascular diseases, and other health issues.

Due to the improved standard of living and the convenience of obtaining food in modern times, coupled with busy work schedules, many people have the habit of having late-night snacks, which also has adverse effects on health.

Eating at night may disrupt the normal digestive process, increase gastric acid secretion, and potentially cause discomfort, heartburn, and gastroesophageal reflux disease.

Late-night snacks often involve high-energy, high-fat, and high-sugar foods, which may contribute to weight gain. The digestion and metabolism of nighttime foods are slower compared to daytime, leading to energy accumulation. In the long run, this may impact insulin sensitivity, increasing the risk of developing diabetes and metabolic syndrome.

Irregular eating times and the consumption of high-fat, high-sugar foods may elevate the risk of cardiovascular diseases. Excessive intake of high-sugar foods can lead to blood sugar fluctuations, increasing the risk of diabetes.

Moreover, overeating, especially consuming caffeine or foods with high calorie content, may affect falling asleep and sleep quality.

Considering these factors collectively, unhealthy lifestyles and poor dietary habits increase the risk of developing cancer, with the gastrointestinal tract being particularly susceptible to cancerous changes due to the digestion and processing of food.

Chapter 3

Briefly How Western Medicine Understands Bowel Cancer

What is bowel cancer?

"Bowel cancer" is a term that is often used interchangeably with "colorectal cancer," which includes cancers that occur in the colon (large intestine) and the rectum. Therefore, colon cancer is a type of bowel cancer, but not all bowel cancers are specifically colon cancer.

The digestive system consists of the small intestine and the large intestine (colon and rectum). Colorectal cancer can develop in either the colon or the rectum. The colon is the upper part of the large intestine, while the rectum is the lower part. The distinction between colon cancer and rectal cancer is based on the location of the cancerous growth.

In summary, colon cancer refers specifically to cancer that originates in the colon (the large intestine).

Rectal cancer refers to cancer that starts in the rectum (the last several inches of the large intestine, connecting the colon to the anus).

Bowel cancer encompasses both colon and rectal cancers, as it refers to cancers that can occur in any part of the large intestine (colon or rectum).

Main Symptoms of Bowel Cancer:

1. Changes in Bowel Habits: Persistent changes in bowel habits are a common early sign of bowel cancer. This may include diarrhea, constipation, or a change in the consistency of stool.

2. Blood in the Stool: Rectal bleeding or the presence of blood in the stool is a significant warning sign. Blood may appear as bright red or darker, tarry stools.

3. Abdominal Discomfort: Persistent abdominal discomfort, such as cramps, gas, bloating, or pain, may occur, especially if it is unrelated to diet or temporary digestive issues.

4. Unexplained Weight Loss: Unintentional weight loss without a clear cause can be a symptom of various cancers, including bowel cancer.

5. Fatigue and Weakness: Bowel cancer can lead to a decrease in the number of red blood cells (anemia), resulting in fatigue, weakness, and pale skin.

6. Incomplete Emptying of Bowels: Feeling that your bowel doesn't empty completely after a bowel movement can be a symptom.

THE SYMPTOMS, DIAGNOSIS, and treatment of colon and rectal cancers are often similar, but some differences may exist based on the specific location within the large intestine. Screening methods, such as colonoscopies, are crucial for early detection and management of both colon and rectal cancers. It's important to consult with a healthcare professional for personalized information and guidance based on an individual's health history and symptoms.

How Western Medicine treats bowel cancer?

Like other western countries, surgery is a primary treatment for bowel cancer in the US. The goal is to remove the tumor along with surrounding tissues and lymph nodes. Depending on the extent of the cancer, surgery may involve removing a portion of the colon or rectum (partial colectomy) or the entire colon (total colectomy).

Chemotherapy is a common method of treatment which involves the use of drugs to kill or slow the growth of cancer cells. It may be administered before surgery (neoadjuvant chemotherapy) to shrink tumors, after surgery (adjuvant chemotherapy) to eliminate any remaining cancer cells, or as the primary treatment for advanced cases.

Another method is radiation therapy that uses high-energy rays to target and destroy cancer cells. It is often used in combination with surgery or chemotherapy, particularly in rectal cancer cases.

Targeted therapy drugs have been developed to target specific molecules involved in cancer growth. They are used in cases where specific genetic mutations or proteins are identified in the cancer cells.

Medications used to treat bowel cancer in Western Medicine

As we discuss above, the treatment of bowel cancer in Western medicine typically involves a multidisciplinary approach, combining surgery, chemotherapy, radiation therapy, and targeted therapy. The specific medications used may vary based on the stage of the cancer, the individual patient's health, and the characteristics of the tumor. Here are some common medications and classes of drugs used in the treatment of bowel cancer:

Chemotherapy Drugs:

Fluorouracil (5-FU): Often used in combination with other drugs, 5-FU is a common chemotherapy medication that interferes with the growth of cancer cells.

Capecitabine: An oral prodrug of 5-FU, capecitabine is often used in the treatment of colorectal cancer.

Oxaliplatin and Irinotecan: These are platinum-based and topoisomerase inhibitor chemotherapy drugs, respectively, frequently used in combination with 5-FU or capecitabine.

Targeted Therapy:

Bevacizumab: A monoclonal antibody that targets vascular endothelial growth factor (VEGF), inhibiting the growth of blood vessels that supply the tumor.

Cetuximab and Panitumumab: Monoclonal antibodies that target the epidermal growth factor receptor (EGFR), blocking signals that promote cancer cell growth.

Immunotherapy:

Nivolumab and Pembrolizumab: Immune checkpoint inhibitors that block the PD-1 protein, allowing the immune system to recognize and attack cancer cells.

Radiation Therapy:

Fluorouracil (5-FU) with Radiation: Sometimes used concurrently with radiation therapy to enhance the treatment's effectiveness.

Surgery:

Surgical procedures involve the removal of the tumor and surrounding tissues. Adjuvant chemotherapy or radiation therapy may follow surgery to target any remaining cancer cells.

The above are only the main medications. It's important to note that the choice of medications and treatment plan is highly individualized and determined by the specific characteristics of the cancer, its stage, and the overall health of the patient.

Chapter 4

Theoretical Basis of TCM In The Treatment Of Bowel Cancer

Chinese Internal Medicine elucidates the etiology, pathogenesis, syndrome characteristics, and principles of differentiation and treatment, as well as the rules for prevention, recovery, and regulation of internal diseases based on TCM theory.

Internal diseases primarily refer to miscellaneous illnesses related to organs, meridians, and fluids as described in "Jin Kui Yao Lue" (Essential Prescriptions of the Golden Coffer) and subsequent internal medicine texts. These conditions, such as diseases of organs and meridians, disorders of qi, blood, body fluids, are mainly caused by internal factors such as emotions, diet, and fatigue. The principles of differentiation and treatment are guided by the theories of organs, meridians, and the physiology and pathology of qi, blood, and body fluids.

Chinese Internal Medicine is divided into various systems, including lung disease patterns, heart and brain disease patterns, spleen and stomach disease patterns, liver and gallbladder disease patterns, kidney and bladder disease patterns, qi, blood, and body fluid disease patterns, and meridian and limb disease patterns. Cancer is also categorized as a separate system within this framework. The occurrence and development of colorectal cancer are closely related to all organ systems, with the most significant connections found in the spleen-stomach system and the large intestine-small intestine, as well as qi, blood, and body fluids.

In addition to diagnosis, it is crucial to focus on understanding the main syndromes and characteristics, etiology, pathogenesis, and treatment principles of colorectal cancer. These aspects constitute the main content of differentiation and treatment in TCM.

Traditional Chinese Medicine (TCM) theory posits that the human body, its various tissues and structures, and the internal functional activities are all in a state of harmonious, coordinated, and balanced "yin-yang equilibrium" with the external environment. If this balance is disrupted due to various internal and external factors, and the body cannot exert its normal physiological functions, disease occurs.

The occurrence of diseases is individualized. Due to the specificity of constitution, individuals may exhibit susceptibility to certain pathogenic factors or diseases. Differences in constitution lead to variations in the interaction between pathogenic and righteous factors, determining different trends in the onset and progression of diseases.

Pathogenic qi is a crucial factor in the development of the majority of internal diseases. Pathogenic qi is categorized into yin and yang and includes internal and external factors, primarily represented by wind, cold, heat, dampness, dryness, and fire. Generally, yang pathogenic factors tend to induce patterns of excess heat, while yin pathogenic factors are more likely to lead to patterns of deficiency cold.

Apart from the six external pathogenic influences, many internal diseases, including cancer, are often caused by imbalances in diet, emotional disturbances, excessive fatigue, and similar factors. These factors gradually lead to disharmony in the organs and the imbalance of qi and blood, resulting in a relatively slow onset of illness.

Illness often originates from the skin and hair, with the onset frequently occurring on the superficial level of the muscles. Emotional factors and dietary imbalances can lead to diseases, typically starting from the disruption of qi and blood, and the organs.

Good behavioral habits are a crucial guarantee of health. The Yellow Emperor's Inner Canon states, "With regulated diet, regular daily life, avoiding overexertion, one can maintain both physical and spiritual well-being and live out their natural lifespan." On the other hand, unhealthy habits, or an unhealthy lifestyle, are significant factors in the onset of internal diseases, especially colorectal cancer.

Regarding the occurrence and progression of internal diseases, common ailments vary with each season. In spring, with windy weather and rising temperatures, wind-related and heat-related diseases are more prevalent. Summer, characterized by hot and rainy conditions, sees an increase in damp-heat and diarrhea-related illnesses. Autumn, marked by dryness and cooler temperatures, sees a rise in dryness-related and respiratory diseases. Winter, being cold, is associated with conditions like kidney deficiency and rheumatic diseases. Colorectal cancer can occur in any season throughout the year.

The onset of internal diseases is closely related to geographical factors. Regions with hot and rainy climates are more prone to damp-heat and warm diseases. Prolonged residence in damp areas increases the likelihood of rheumatic and obstructive diseases. Colorectal cancer is associated with damp-heat syndrome.

Abnormal eating habits refer to a symptom where a patient experiences changes in appetite and food intake, commonly observed in various internal diseases, with a particular prevalence in disorders related to the spleen and stomach. The underlying pathology is often the dysfunction and disruption of digestive functions in the spleen and stomach. Conditions such as colitis or cancer in the colon can directly lead to abnormal eating habits, and the two may also mutually exacerbate each other.

For instance, symptoms such as poor appetite, fullness and discomfort in the epigastric region, accompanied by a slimy tongue coating and a slippery pulse, indicate dampness obstruction. Yellowing of the complexion, loose or watery stools, reduced appetite, and abdominal distension suggest a combination of spleen deficiency and dampness.

Abnormalities in bowel movements refer to deviations in the frequency, characteristics, and color of stool from the usual, often indicative of symptoms related to the spleen and stomach systems. They can also reflect the body's state of cold or heat, as well as the abundance or decline of bodily qi, blood, and fluids. The basic pathology of abnormal bowel movements is various factors leading to irregular bowel transit, which is common in colitis and colorectal cancer.

For instance, dry and difficult-to-pass stools, accompanied by a dry mouth, red tongue, and scanty saliva, suggest a condition of Yin deficiency and intestinal dryness. An increase in the frequency of bowel movements with watery stools resembling water indicates excessive dampness or diarrhea due to spleen deficiency. Yellow, mushy, and foul-smelling stools are indicative of damp-heat-induced diarrhea, while a feeling of incomplete bowel emptying, urgency, and heaviness may suggest damp-heat obstruction.

Incomplete digestion of grains in stool is often due to spleen deficiency and inadequate digestive function. If the stool has a foul odor and is accompanied by abdominal distension and pain, it may be attributed to impaired digestion.

White stools, along with jaundice in the body and eyes, accompanied by itching, suggest the stagnation of damp-heat in the liver and gallbladder. Stool with pus and blood is a sign of dysentery. Stool that is black like tar indicates distant bleeding in the gastrointestinal tract, often associated with stomach and intestinal damage. Stool with fresh red blood indicates bleeding closer to the anus, commonly seen in conditions such as heat damaging the intestines, blood stasis, or blood-heat obstructing the intestines, as well as hemorrhoids.

The color of rectal bleeding can be indicative of its location. Black stool suggests bleeding from the upper gastrointestinal tract, termed distant bleeding. Fresh blood in the stool or blood after initially passing stool suggests bleeding from the lower segment of the intestine or hemorrhoids, termed near bleeding.

Generally, a gradual reduction in the frequency of bowel movements, a transition from loose to soft stools, and a change from black to yellow stools signify a positive progression of the illness. Conversely, an increase in bowel movements, a shift from soft to loose stools, and a change from yellow to black stools indicate a worsening condition. If, during a severe stage of the illness, there is a sudden loss of bowel control and a drastic increase in bowel movements, it may be an indication of sinking of yang qi, requiring special attention.

Typically, diseases progress from mild to severe, from relatively simple to complex interconnections. In the early stages of the disease, when the body's righteous qi is relatively strong, early treatment can yield better therapeutic effects and alleviate the patient's suffering more quickly. As the disease advances, becoming more complex and variable, with the interplay of deficiency and excess, cold and heat, it poses many challenges to treatment and may even lead to serious consequences.

"Treating what is urgent when the urgent symptoms occur" refers to the principle in the development of a disease that, if there are critical and life-threatening symptoms affecting the patient's safety, it is necessary to prioritize the resolution of these critical symptoms.

"Treat the root causes when a disease has developed in a gradual manner" refers to the general principle of treating diseases that evolve relatively steadily or chronic illnesses.

"Supporting the Righteous and Expelling the Pathogenic" is one of the important principles in the treatment of internal diseases in Traditional Chinese Medicine (TCM). "Supporting the Righteous" involves using treatment methods such as nourishing qi, replenishing blood, nourishing yin, and reinforcing yang to support and supplement the body's righteous qi. "Expelling the Pathogenic" involves using methods such as inducing sweating, purging, resolving dampness, promoting diuresis, promoting bowel movements, and resolving blood stasis to eliminate and eradicate the pathogenic factors causing the disease.

Treatment should be tailored to the individual. Based on the patient's gender, age, constitution, and other characteristics, the principle of considering the individual in treatment is followed, known as

"Tailoring Treatment to the Individual." For example, considering the physiological characteristics related to menstruation, pregnancy, and postpartum in women is essential. Different ages come with variations in physiological functions and disease characteristics. Elderly individuals may exhibit blood and qi deficiencies, reduced organ function, and are more prone to deficiency patterns or cases with a combination of deficiency and excess. The treatment approach for deficiency patterns involves tonifying, while caution is required when dealing with excess patterns to avoid harming the righteous qi. Different constitutions may vary in strength, predisposition to cold or heat, and the presence of pre-existing conditions. Therefore, even if suffering from the same illness, treatment approaches may need to be different, such as being cautious with warm tonics for individuals with a hot constitution and avoiding cold remedies for those with a cold constitution.

Traditional Chinese Medicine (TCM) employs various methods for the treatment of colorectal cancer, and important approaches include heat-clearing, purgative, harmonizing, warming the interior, resolving, regulating blood, and tonifying methods.

Heat-clearing method, also known as "Qing Fa," involves the use of cold or cool herbs with heat-clearing properties to treat diseases with a heat syndrome.

Purgative method, also known as "Xia Fa," involves promoting bowel movements, eliminating accumulation, purging excess, and expelling dampness to dispel pathogenic factors. This method is widely applied to conditions involving dry feces, stagnation, excess heat, and water retention.

Harmonizing method aims to treat pathological changes between the surface and interior, as well as among the organs, through harmonizing and coordinating therapeutic approaches.

Warming the interior method, also known as "Wen Fa," uses warm or hot herbs to dispel cold pathogenic factors and tonify yang qi.

Resolving method, also known as "Xiao Fa," involves resolving and dispersing accumulated pathogenic factors, gradually dissipating accumulated and stagnant substances. This method is also known as "to remove or get rid of the evils."

Regulating blood method involves adjusting the circulation of blood to treat blood stasis and various bleeding disorders.

Tonifying method, also known as "Bu Fa," utilizes herbs with tonifying properties to treat deficiencies in yin, yang, qi, blood, fluids, and organs. This method is widely applicable to various deficiency syndromes.

These methods collectively form an integral part of TCM's comprehensive approach to treating colorectal cancer, taking into account the specific nature and manifestations of the individual patient's condition.

Chapter 5

My Experience Of Treating Ulcerative Colitis Can Be Applied To Bowel Cancer Treatment

In order to cure my ulcerative colitis, I researched deep into the root of bowel cancer. Here I would like to share more on my study of the disease.

Zheng Qin'an, a physician of the Fuyang school, said in "Yifayuantong"(Treatment Methods and Ideas): "For those with chronic illness or inherently insufficient strength, if they suddenly suffer from unstoppable bleeding in their stools, this indicates that the lower jiao lacks fire and cannot control it, leading to a potential prolapse. It is urgent to administer large doses of yang-restoring treatments, such as Fuzi Lizhong and Huiyang Drink." The thought of the Fuyang school once influenced my medication, but after all, my condition was not severe enough to require yang-restoring treatment for prolapse. I tried to use yang to treat bleeding, but the effect was not ideal.

Dr. Zhu Danxi's "Collection of My Clinical Methods" states, "For bleeding, it is not advisable to use purely cold and cool medicines; it is necessary to add pungent flavors to assist in these cold medicines. For those who do not heal over time, later use warm remedies, must also be uplifting, add wine-soaked and stir-fried cool medicines, and cook with wine Coptis pills and the like, because it's a case of cold induced by heat." Zhu Danxi's idea of using pungent flavors as an adjunct made me disregard foods like chili peppers in my diet for a while, which led to a recurrence of my condition.

Chen Xiuyuan, a medical expert, gives a detailed description of treating dysentery. In his "Miao Yong Shi Fang" (Wonderful Use of Seasonal Prescriptions), he discusses the treatment methods for several main symptoms. For example, "If there is fever without aversion to cold and a sense of urgency and heaviness in the rectum, use Ge Gen (Kudzu Root) Huang Qin (Scutellaria) Huang Lian (Coptis) Gan Cao (Licorice) Decoction. According to the ancient method, first decoct Ge Gen, then the other medicines, take two to three doses a day, and you will surely recover." He also said, "According to its treatment method, it is nothing more than using substances like E Jiao (Donkey-hide gelatin), Di Yu (Garden Burnet), Huai Hua (Pagoda Tree Flower), and Cang Zhu (Atractylodes), how can it be used to save a critical condition. If there is fresh blood in the diarrhea, thirst, short urine, urgency and heaviness in the rectum, and a strong pulse, it is a fire syndrome, suitable for Bai Tou Weng Tang (Pulsatilla Decoction), take twice a day." He also said, "If the spleen and stomach are weak, it is appropriate to use Xiang Sha Liu Jun Zi Tang and Li Zhong Tang to strengthen the spleen and stomach." This seems to be an ancient general treatment method, which I have tried one by one, sometimes with good and bad effects. But I firmly believe that it is a problem of my own lack of proficiency, not a problem with traditional Chinese medicine itself.

Yu Chang, a Qing Dynasty medical expert, said that in treating dysentery, "you must first resolve the exterior, then regulate the interior. First use pungent-cool to resolve the exterior, then use bitter-cold to clear the interior." "The stomach is affected by damp-heat, and the food and drink are transformed by the fire of the Shaoyang into filth, which then enters the large intestine. Treating only the Yangming and not the Shaoyang is useless. The qi of Shaoyang, which generates and transmits, enters the earth and thus sinks. If you do not first lift it with pungent-cool and directly snatch it away with bitter-cold, the dysentery will never end." I studied Yu Chang's book relatively late, but Yu Chang's statement really gets to the root of the problem.

The book "Nei Jing Ji Yao" (Key Points of Huangdi Neijing) says: "If there is heaviness behind, it is appropriate to purge; if there is abdominal pain, it is appropriate to harmonize; if there is body heaviness, remove dampness; if there is a taut pulse, eliminate wind; if there is thick and sticky pus and blood, use heavy doses to deplete it; if there is body cold with spontaneous sweating, use hot medicine to warm it; if there is an internal blockage of wind-evil, it is appropriate to induce sweating; if there is diarrhea with undigested food, it is appropriate to warm it."

According to Zhongjing's treatment for dysentery, Cheng Qi Tang (Tangerine Peel Decoction) is used for cases that can be purged. The cold nature of Da Huang (Rhubarb) is good at moving, assisted by the warmth of Hou Po (Magnolia Bark), which is good at moving stagnant qi. Moderated by the sweetness of Gan Cao (Licorice) and taken with the decoction, it irrigates and cleanses the intestines and stomach, moisturizes and lightens, and stops accumulations. Indeed, this is so. I spent ten years understanding the nuances of this.

My ulcerative colitis, in terms of its etiology and pathogenesis, is no different from bloody dysentery, both being caused by damp-heat. The lungs transfer heat to the large intestine, where the heat evil resides inside, rushing to the large intestine and stagnating in the bladder, hindering the transformation of qi.

Due to my prolonged dysentery, the pathogen entered the yin, occasionally leading to heat from yin deficiency. The heat, unceasing, causes the condition to recur. The treatment should follow the Nei Jing's universal method of guiding heat downward, clearing the heat in the bladder, and facilitating the movement of qi. First use pungent-cool to release the exterior, then use bitter-cold to clear the interior, guiding external pathogens out from the interior. Apart from this, there is no other effective method.

Why should Da Huang Tang (Rhubarb Decoction) be decocted with two cups of wine? Because wine-processed Da Huang can enhance its blood-activating effect and also reduce the coldness of Da Huang.

Ancient medical texts record that Da Huang is slightly toxic, while modern texts say it is non-toxic; apart from wine, adding a bit of Gan Cao can also neutralize the toxicity of Da Huang. Generally, wine-processed Da Huang uses rice wine, like Shaoxing rice wine. I used fine Australian Penfolds wine, and the effect was equally good.

In the process of exploring treatment methods, I once overused purgatives, leading to chest congestion or spleen deficiency, which then needed to be treated with substances like Shen Ling Bai Zhu and others to recuperate. Or sometimes, my diet was not disciplined. Thus, this condition of mine relapsed and recurred four or five times over ten years. What is the reason for the recurrence after recovery?

According to the Inner Canon, those who rest from dysentery do so intermittently; sometimes it stops and then recurs. This may be because the pathogenic qi has not been completely dispelled and suddenly stops, then recurs. Or it could be due to indulging in rich flavors right after recovery, or engaging in reckless physical exertion, all of which can cause a relapse.

The "Jin Gui Yao Lue" (Essential Prescriptions from the Golden Cabinet) states: "If diarrhea has ceased but recurs on specific years, months, days, or hours, it is because the illness has not been completely resolved. It should be treated with purgation, and Da Cheng Qi Tang (Major Order the Qi Decoction) is appropriate. For those with intermittent dysentery, where it stops but does not completely cease, and the righteous qi is already weak while the pathogen is not fully eliminated, purgation should not be immediately considered. In such cases, the illness has been stopped for a long time, the righteous qi has recovered, but the accumulation has not been removed. Therefore, it is necessary to purge."

Having decided on the purgative method, Da Huang (Rhubarb) is the main herb. During the initial period of taking the medicine, there may be an increase in the amount of blood or sticky substances, indicating that the damp-heat has not been completely cleared.

Sometimes the urine may appear nearly red-yellow, which is the color of Da Huang itself and should not cause fear. One should continue to clear the internal heat until there is no pain in the anus during or after bowel movements. After the heat and toxins are fully cleared, use medicines like Shao Yao Tang (Peony Decoction) to harmonize Shaoyang, nourishing yin and blood with yin-tonifying herbs, and use Shen Ling Bai Zhu Wan (Ginseng, Poria, and Atractylodes Pill) to support the righteous qi.

When studying ancient Chinese medical text, learners should not attach themselves to the exact words or characters, they should reach out to the idea, meaning or philosophy behind those words.

I hope that my journey to curing ulcerative colitis would serve as a guidance for other physicians who have the desire to find better solutions for cancer treatment related to the colon and the bowel.

Chapter 6

Discussion on Treatment of Cancers

In 1964, a Chinese doctor successfully performed the first bone marrow transplant surgery on a leukemia (blood cancer) patient using her identical twin sister as the donor. In the 1970s and 80s, Lu Daopei was the first to go to various European countries to study and learn about the treatment of leukemia. He later founded a hematological hospital in Beijing and achieved remarkable success in the fields of immunotherapy and bone marrow transplantation.

However, matching bone marrow types is very difficult. Leukemia can recur after a bone marrow transplant, and although the patient's condition may improve, the cure rate is very low. This is currently the best treatment method in Western medicine.

Cancer is a general term for a variety of malignant tumors, characterized by abnormal proliferation of visceral and tissue. The proliferating masses often occur in combination with qi stagnation, phlegm coagulation, damp stagnation, blood stasis, and accumulation of toxins, eventually forming tangible tumors over time. Cancer patients often have a weak constitution, and the cancerous lesions consume the body's qi, blood, and body fluids, leading to changes in the disease mechanism such as deficiency of qi and blood, and deficiency of both yin and yang in the middle and late stages of the disease.

In traditional Chinese medicine, there is no concept of "cancer." The corresponding disease is called "◇◇" ◇accumulation and gathering into masses). Since the concept of "cancer" has been widely accepted, we refer to it as cancer for the time being.

The "Nan Jing: Article 55" states: Accumulation (◇) is yin qi, while gathering (◇) is yang qi. Therefore, yin is deep and latent, yang is superficial and active. Where qi accumulates, it is called accumulation; where qi gathers, it is called gathering. Thus, accumulations are generated by the five viscera; gatherings are formed by the six fu organs. Accumulation is yin qi; it starts in a fixed location, its pain does not stray from its area, it has definite starting and ending points vertically, and limited extent horizontally. Gathering is yang qi; it starts without a fixed root, does not stay in a specific area vertically, and its pain does not have a constant location, which is called gathering. Thus, this is how to distinguish between accumulation and gathering.

In "Ling Shu: Unchanging," Emperor Huangdi asks: How can one diagnose accumulations and gatherings in the intestines? His Imperial Physician Qiao Yu answers: If the skin is thin and not lustrous, and the flesh is not firm but soggy. In such cases, the intestines and stomach are averse; when there is aversion, pathogenic qi stays, and accumulation and gathering then damage the area between the spleen and stomach. If cold and heat are irregular, pathogenic qi gradually arrives. When accumulation and stagnation persist, a major gathering arises.

"Yi Lin Gai Cuo" says: No matter where, there is always blood and qi. Qi is formless and cannot form masses. Masses must be formed from tangible blood. Blood, when cold, coagulates into masses; when heated, it is simmered into masses.

Cancer is formed on the basis of an imbalance in the yin and yang, qi and blood of the viscera and bowels, with the invasion of the six excesses (pathogenic factors) and toxins, combining with qi, phlegm, dampness, stasis, and heat to form accumulations. The overall mechanism of the disease is that of a weak foundation with excess symptoms; the weak foundation refers to the deficiency of qi, blood, yin, and yang of the viscera and bowels, while the excess symptoms are the mutual entanglement of qi stagnation, phlegm turbidity, blood stasis, and heat toxins, forming masses.

Tumor specialist Qian Bowen believes that tumor diseases are local manifestations of a systemic disease, closely related to the whole body. Therefore, the key to effective treatment lies in the dialectical application of supporting the healthy energy and eliminating the pathogenic factors. Traditionally, treatment of tumors generally focuses on attacking the pathogen in the early stage, combining attack and support in the mid-stage, and primarily supporting the healthy energy in the late stage. However, Qian Bowen does not adhere to this rule rigidly; he believes that support should be provided in the early stages and attacking the pathogen should also be considered in the late stages, depending on the actual situation of the disease, the severity, and urgency, and balancing attack and support. Especially in treating late-stage patients, one must not be rigid in focusing only on support; it is essential to include elements of draining in the support and elements of support in the draining, meaning that supporting the healthy energy should be combined with anti-cancer treatment.

We often hear from Western medicine that cancer requires "early detection and early treatment." Early treatment typically refers to rapid surgical removal, chemotherapy, electrotherapy, and radiation therapy, which is extremely misguided. Cancer patients often do not die from the tumor itself, but from the damage caused by medical surgery to the human body, and from the inflammation prevention treatment after surgery. The further damage to the heart and kidneys due to inflammation prevention is often the real cause of death for these patients.

Dr. Ni Haixia attempted to treat leukemia using traditional Chinese medicine methods, claiming satisfactory results with remedies like Si Ni Tang (Frigid Extremities Decoction). He believes that leukemia is a case of true cold and false heat, a symptom of reversed qi. The transformation of red blood cells to white is closely related to the liver.

It is important to note that after chemotherapy, a patient's blood vessels become as rigid and hard as plastic pipes. This hardening of the blood vessels leads to circulatory obstacles, increasing the load on the heart. The damage caused by chemical drugs can lead to the failure of the heart and kidneys. Thus, it is the medical treatment that causes death, not the disease itself.

Medical expert Zhang Zhaohan states that abnormal cancerous tumors, caused by bodily harm and insufficient thermal energy, are similar to whitening hair and wrinkled skin; they are natural phenomena that occur in the process of life's deterioration and aging, and are not necessarily fatal diseases. Unfortunately, patients, not knowing the truth, undergo examinations and end up with exaggerated and vilified diagnoses. Some doctors even claim that without surgery and chemotherapy, the tumor will worsen, and the patient has only a few years to live. This fear instilled in patients is the true beginning of a nightmare.

Dr. Peng Yijun from Taiwan said, "When a doctor tells you that surgery is the only and necessary treatment option, you might only hear a warning not to undergo the surgery if you wish to live longer, especially if you have a relative or close friend working as a physician in that hospital. Why is this? Today's medical science and the experiences of patients can be described as one of the most tragic, cruel, and darkest eras in medical history. The general public's understanding of diseases is perhaps the most distorted, impoverished, ignorant, and fearful. Why has human health suffered such a catastrophe?"

The doctor who had 30 years experience in Western Medicine criticized the general practice of Western Medicine on the treatment of cancers, stating, "One of the astonishing advancements of modern medicine is the creation of cancer, which now ranks first on the top ten list of causes of death. Currently, one in four patients dies from cancer. The medical scams that lead patients to financial ruin and family destruction are becoming more sophisticated, leaving patients with no room for complaint or resistance."

"In cancer treatment, we often hear and see that the 'only' treatment method is early detection and early treatment, including rapid surgical removal, chemotherapy, radiotherapy, and radiation treatment. In reality, these 'only' scientific methods – surgery, chemotherapy, radiotherapy, radiation treatment, and removal – are often the true culprits in prematurely ending patients' lives."

"One can observe the blood vessels of patients who have undergone chemotherapy, which become as hard and rigid as plastic pipes. This hardening of the blood vessels leads to circulatory obstructions, which increase the burden on the heart. Combined with the damage from chemical drugs, this often results in death due to heart and kidney failure, caused by the treatment rather than the disease itself."

Dr. Peng raised an alarming question, "Cancer surgery and removal do not signify the success of medical treatment, but rather mark the beginning of another period of pain and sorrow for the patient. Can cancer cells be completely eradicated?"

The following discussion is based on "◇◇◇◇◇"◇TCM Internal Medicine◇published in 2017 by China TCM Press and used by Chinese TCM universities as textbook.

Analysis of the Causes of Various Cancers

THE ONSET OF CANCER is multifaceted, with the main pathogenic mechanisms as follows:

Qi Stagnation: This primarily affects the pulse and organ or corresponding areas, manifesting as distension, pain, a thin and greasy tongue coating, and a taut pulse. The characteristic symptoms of qi stagnation include distension and pain, often characterized by distending pain rather than sharp pain. The pain can move around and come and go intermittently.

Phlegm Coagulation: The main symptoms include cough with phlegm, confusion, phlegm masses, joint pain, lumps in the affected organs, a white tongue coating, and a slippery pulse. The characteristic signs of turbid phlegm in the lungs include cough with expectoration, while phlegm clouding the mind leads to confusion and incoherent speech. Phlegm stagnating in muscles and bones results in phlegm masses. When phlegm blocks the meridians, it causes joint pain. Phlegm congealing in the organs, often intertwined with dampness or blood stasis, leads to lumps that are not hard and may be painful.

Damp Stagnation: The main symptoms include cough with phlegm, poor appetite, dullness, abdominal distension, diarrhea, difficulty in urination, a white greasy or slippery tongue coating, and a soggy pulse. The characteristic signs include dampness stagnating in the upper burner causing cough with expectoration, in the middle burner leading to poor appetite, dullness, abdominal distension, diarrhea, and in the lower burner causing difficulty in urination.

Blood Stasis: The main symptoms include pain in the affected area, fixed pain, bruises or lumps, fever, a dark complexion, abnormal skin and nails, a dark purplish tongue, or spots on the tongue, and a choppy or taut pulse. The characteristic symptom of blood stasis is pain, often fixed and piercing, persisting for a long time, and recurring.

Toxic Accumulation: The main symptoms include fever, bleeding, redness, swelling, heat, pain in the affected area, constipation, dark, scanty urine, a red tongue with a yellow coating, and a rapid pulse. The characteristic sign of toxicity, being an extreme form of fire, is marked by prominent signs of heat.

Syndromes of Cancers

THE MAIN SYNDROMES of cancers are as follows:

Qi Deficiency: The main symptoms include listlessness, fatigue, shortness of breath, dizziness, spontaneous sweating, susceptibility to colds, pale complexion, a pale tongue, thin white tongue coating, and a weak pulse. The characteristic features are a series of symptoms indicating depletion of vital energy and reduced organ function. Symptoms vary depending on the affected organ.

Blood Deficiency: The main symptoms include dizziness, fatigue, insomnia, forgetfulness, palpitations, pale or sallow complexion, unmoistened lips and nails, a pale tongue, white tongue coating, and a weak pulse. The features of this syndrome are a series of symptoms indicating malnourishment due to blood deficiency and reduced organ function. The main difference from qi deficiency is the prominent signs of blood and nutrient deficiency, such as a lackluster complexion and unmoistened lips and nails, often accompanied by excessive blood loss.

Yin Deficiency: The main symptoms include dry mouth and lips, irritability with a sensation of heat in the chest, palms, and soles, night sweats, restlessness, insomnia, weakness in the lumbar and knees, dry skin, constipation, a red tongue with little moisture, and a fine, rapid pulse. The features of this syndrome are a series of symptoms indicating a deficiency of yin fluids and a loss of moistening and cooling functions. Yin deficiency often generates internal heat, commonly accompanied by signs of false heat.

Yang Deficiency: The main symptoms include lethargy, a desire to lie down, shortness of breath and disinclination to speak, cold limbs, palpitations, spontaneous sweating, poor appetite, edema of the limbs, pale or sallow complexion, cold pain in the lumbar region and knees, impotence or spermatorrhea, loose stools, long clear urination, a pale and swollen tongue with tooth marks, white tongue coating, and a deep, slow pulse. The features of this syndrome are a series of symptoms indicating a deficiency of yang energy and a loss of warming and activating functions. Yang deficiency leads to internal cold, often marked by signs of false cold.

The Pathogenesis of Cancers

HERE IS A SUMMARY OF the pathogenesis of various cancers:

1.**Qi Stagnation**: Emotional distress, dietary imbalances, exposure to external pathogens, as well as obstruction caused by phlegm-dampness and blood stasis, can all lead to qi stagnation. This stagnation impedes the flow of qi and blood, causing swelling and pain in the affected organs or body parts.

2.**Phlegm Coagulation**: Caused by external factors or internal injuries, phlegm coagulation occurs when the lungs fail to distribute fluids properly, the spleen fails to transport and transform fluids, and the kidneys fail to warm and vaporize fluids, leading to the internal generation of turbid phlegm. Depending on the affected area, this can manifest in various clinical symptoms, with coughing up phlegm, phlegm nodules, and lumps being characteristic.

3.**Damp Stagnation**: Caused by external factors or internal injuries, damp stagnation arises when the functions of the lungs, spleen, and kidneys are disrupted, leading to metabolic disorders of body fluids and the accumulation of dampness. This can manifest in various ways depending on the affected area, with symptoms such as poor appetite, dullness, abdominal distension, and diarrhea, especially when the dampness affects the spleen and stomach.

4.**Blood Stasis**: Emotional distress, dietary imbalances, external pathogens, physical trauma, and chronic illness leading to overall weakness can all cause blood stasis. This condition is characterized by impeded blood flow and, in more severe cases, blocked vessels, leading to pain, fever from congestion, and over time, the formation of masses. This chapter highlights the formation of masses as a prominent feature.

5.**Toxin Accumulation**: Caused by external heat pathogens or internally generated pathogenic factors like phlegm coagulation, damp stagnation, and blood stasis, these can obstruct the flow of qi, leading to prolonged heat or the combination of internal and external pathogens, resulting in excessive heat or 'toxin.' This excessive heat can cause fever, reckless movement of blood leading to bleeding, and the formation of masses due to the accumulation of phlegm, dampness, and blood stasis.

6.**Qi Deficiency**: This is primarily due to dietary imbalances, inadequate nourishment from food essence, or insufficient sources of Qi. It can also result from severe or prolonged illness, weakness in old age, or excessive fatigue. This leads to weakened organ function and inadequate generation of Qi. Due to insufficient vital energy, the body cannot perform its functions of movement, securing, warming, and protecting against external factors, resulting in symptoms like fatigue, listlessness, spontaneous sweating, and susceptibility to colds.

7. **Blood Deficiency**: Often caused by excessive blood loss, weakness of the spleen and stomach, poor nutrition, chronic illness, or disorders in blood generation. Due to the deficiency of nutritive blood, organs and meridians are inadequately nourished, leading to symptoms such as dizziness, fatigue, a pale complexion, and lackluster nails and lips.

8. **Yin Deficiency**: This may result from dry-heat damaging the Yin, or long-term illness affecting the Kidney's primordial Yin. Due to the depletion of Yin essence, the body loses its ability to nourish and moisturize organs, meridians, and bones, causing symptoms like dry mouth, dry lips, dry skin, etc. Yin deficiency leads to excess Yang, manifesting in symptoms of irritability, a sensation of heat in the chest, palms, and soles, night sweats, and other signs of false heat.

9. **Yang Deficiency**: Often a further development of Qi deficiency, where the depletion of Qi affects Yang energy. Due to the decline of Yang Qi, the body loses its warming and invigorating functions, leading to symptoms such as lethargy, desire to sleep, shortness of breath, reluctance to speak, cold limbs, and other signs of cold deficiency.

Key Points to Ponder in Cancer Treatment

CANCER IS CONSIDERED a disease characterized by a deficiency in vital energy and an excess of pathogenic factors, where the pathogen is strong, and the body's natural defenses are weak. Therefore, the basic principle of treatment is to support the body's natural defenses while eliminating pathogenic factors, applying both strengthening and attacking strategies.

Treatment should be based on a comprehensive analysis of the patient's medical history, disease progression, combined with four-diagnostic methods and laboratory tests. It is essential to balance treating the pathogenic factors while considering the body's weaknesses, and to strengthen the body without neglecting the treatment of the pathogenic factors. The methods to support the body's natural defenses mainly depend on the type of deficiency (Qi, Blood, Yin, or Yang) and the main affected organ, using appropriate methods to supplement Qi, Blood, Yin, or Yang. To eliminate pathogenic factors, treatments typically focus on regulating Qi, resolving phlegm, dispelling masses, invigorating blood, removing blood stasis, clearing heat, and detoxifying.

During treatment, methods to invigorate blood, resolve phlegm, disperse masses, and regulate Qi are often used. At the same time, medicines that supplement Qi, Blood, Yin, and Yang are also employed to strengthen the body's defenses against pathogenic factors.

Additionally, external treatment methods such as warm compresses and massage may be used depending on the patient's condition. Strengthening dietary care, regulating emotions, and ensuring adequate rest are also beneficial for the recovery from cancer.

To learn more about the diagnosis and recommended herbs used in cancer treatment, please refer to my book "Every Person Is Their Own Best Doctor - Traditional Chinese Medicine In Practice" or my Chinese book for a more comprehensive and in-depth study.

Chapter 7

Ancient Chinese physicians' Analysis Of The Etiology Of Bowel Cancer

Let's discuss the ancient Chinese medicine's analysis of the etiology of colorectal cancer. In traditional Chinese medicine (TCM), there is no specific term for "colorectal cancer." Analyzing its occurrence and clinical features, it would fall within the categories of TCM diseases such as "intestinal accumulation," "accumulation and stagnation," "zheng jia" (masses or lumps in the abdomen), "intestine stagnation," "intestinal wind," "toxic accumulation in the organs," "diarrhea," and "anal sphincter obstruction" or "hemorrhoids."

About "intestine stagnation", the imperial physician Qibo who served Emperor Huangdi, stated in "Ling Shu Jing" : "Cold qi invades the exterior of the intestines, conflicting with the wei qi (defensive qi); then, polyps are formed. In the beginning, they are as small as chicken eggs, gradually enlarging until fully developed, resembling the state of carrying a child. Over time, they harden, becoming firm to touch and can be displaced with pressure."

The description of these symptoms closely resembles the manifestation of intra-abdominal masses seen in colorectal cancer.

The medical expert Chao Yuanfang from the Sui Dynasty recorded in "Zhu Bing Yuan Hou Lun" (Treatise on the Origin and Symptoms of Diseases): "The disease arises from the disorder of cold and warm, leading to the weakness of the qi in the organs. When food and drink are not digested, they accumulate internally, gradually forming masses that grow over time and do not move due to exhaustion. This condition is referred to as a disease. The description of its form can be verified and examined."

This record helps in understanding the etiology, symptoms, and signs of colorectal cancer.

The Ming Dynasty medical practitioner Chen Shigong, in his work "Wai Ke Zheng Zong" (Orthodox Manual of External Medicine), stated: "Toxins accumulate in the organs, and fiery heat flows towards the anus. The accumulation results in swelling, causing continuous pain in the lower abdomen. The anus feels heavy, and there is a disharmony in bowel movements, either diarrhea or constipation. The anus corrodes internally, eroding through the meridians, allowing contaminated fluids to flow through large openings. Despite an intense thirst, the individual refrains from eating. All these symptoms may occur without the manifestation of the actual disease."

This description outlines the similar etiology, key symptoms, and explicitly indicates a poor prognosis, resembling characteristics associated with colorectal cancer.

In the Qing Dynasty medical text "Wai Ke Da Cheng," it is discussed regarding hemorrhoids: "Suo Gan Zhi (literally translated as 'locked anal hemorrhoids') makes the anus tight both internally and externally, resembling the tightness of bamboo joints or the appearance of a jellyfish. There is urgency with a sensation of heaviness in the rectum. The stool becomes thin and flattened, occasionally accompanied by the discharge of foul-smelling fluids. This condition is incurable."

The description of these symptoms closely aligns with those associated with rectal cancer.

According to traditional Chinese medicine, the large intestine includes the ileum and the rectum. The ileum connects to the cecum at its upper end and to the rectum at its lower end, with the rectum ending at the anus. Its meridians are linked to the lungs and are governed by the spleen. Its physiological function is to receive the turbid matter passed down from the small intestine, further absorb the fluids, oversee the transmission of waste, and excrete it from the body.

The occurrence of colorectal cancer is attributed to the internal factor of deficiency in vital energy (Zheng Qi) and the external factor of the invasion of pathogenic toxins, with both factors influencing each other. A deficiency in vital energy makes the body susceptible to the invasion of pathogenic toxins, which further damages the vital energy. Moreover, when the vital energy is weakened, it lacks the strength to resist the pathogenic factors, leading to their retention. Qi stagnation, blood stasis, and the retention of toxins in the large intestine cause obstruction and accumulation, leading to the loss of functional regulation in the large intestine. Over time, this accumulation develops internally and manifests as colorectal cancer.

Prolonged residence in damp environments or exposure to external dampness can lead to the invasion of damp evils. This invasion causes the stagnation of dampness in the spleen, resulting in a weakened spleen function. As a consequence, both internal and external dampness persist over time, potentially triggering the onset of this condition.

Irregular dietary habits, excessive consumption of greasy and rich foods, indulgence in alcoholic beverages and dairy products, or overconsumption of raw and cold foods can all damage the spleen and stomach. This damage fosters the production of dampness, which, when not properly transformed and eliminated, may accumulate and exert pressure on the large intestine. The interaction between this accumulated dampness and intestinal waste can lead to obstruction, impact, or the gradual formation of toxins, damaging the intestines and evolving into the present condition.

Emotional disturbances, unfulfilled desires, or emotional injuries can result in liver qi stagnation. When the liver wood overacts and restrains the spleen earth, the spleen's healthy functioning is compromised. This disturbance leads to the internal generation of water and dampness. The stagnation transforms into heat, and the combination of damp-heat pathology can exert pressure on the large intestine, potentially giving rise to this condition.

In individuals with weakened vital energy due to congenital deficiencies or age-related physical decline, there is often a deficiency in both the spleen and kidneys. The kidneys represent the foundation of congenital energy, while the spleen serves as the foundation for acquired energy. The relationship between these two organs and the transformation of water and dampness is closely connected. When both organs are deficient, it leads to internal retention of water and dampness, which, over time, can contribute to the onset of this condition.

While the disease is located in the intestines, its relationship with the spleen, stomach, liver, and kidneys is particularly significant. In the early stages, the pathology is primarily characterized by damp-heat and stagnant toxic evils. In the later stages, it often involves a combination of deficiency in righteous qi and the presence of pathogenic evils. Deficiency in righteous qi commonly manifests as spleen-kidney qi deficiency, spleen-kidney yang deficiency, deficiency in both qi and blood, and liver-kidney yin deficiency. External exposure to damp-heat or damage to the spleen and stomach leading to the internal generation of water and dampness, coupled with prolonged stagnation transforming into heat, is a crucial factor in the development of the disease.

The prolonged presence of damp-heat obstructs the intestines, hinders the flow of qi, and the heat gradually transforms into toxins, damaging the meridians and leading to the accumulation of qi stagnation, damp-heat, toxins, and blood stasis in the intestines. This constitutes the main pathological process underlying the onset of the disease.

The "Huangdi Neijing" states that when the nourishing qi (Rong Qi) fails to circulate properly and goes against the flesh and tendons, it gives rise to the formation of abscesses and swellings. Changes in the richness of diet can lead to the emergence of large carbuncles, as if the nourishing qi is being held back by emptiness. The dampness in the earth's qi can harm the skin, flesh, tendons, and meridians.

Li Dongyuan, a medical expert from the Song Dynasty, explained that when dampness externally injures the body, the nourishing qi fails to circulate. The functions of nourishment and defense are carried out by the qi associated with the spleen and stomach. The spleen qi is responsible for moving the qi. The nourishing qi is fundamental, and when its proper circulation is obstructed by dampness, it leads to the formation of sores and ulcers. Similarly, the changes resulting from an excessive and rich diet are also explained. It refers to the consumption of concentrated and rich flavors, causing the nourishing qi to move against its natural direction, condensing in the meridians and resulting in the formation of sores and ulcers.

The Ming Dynasty physician Wang Kentang discussed the origins of abscesses and ulcers, stating, "There are five sources for the formation of abscesses and ulcers. First, the atmospheric qi changing with the seasons. Second, internal stagnation caused by the Seven Emotions. Third, weakness in the body and external exposure to pathogenic factors. Fourth, internal heat struggling against cold wind. Fifth, the consumption of excessively hot and toxic substances, such as spicy and fried foods, alcoholic beverages, and the intake of medicinal substances with heat toxicity."

Gao Bingjun, a physician from the Qing Dynasty, believed that the occurrence of abscesses in the large intestine may be attributed to various factors. Individuals who regularly indulge in strong alcoholic beverages and spicy foods might generate damp-heat, leading to stagnation and damage to the lungs, preventing the proper dispersion and descent of lung qi. This can result in the downward flow of damp-heat, obstructing the circulation of qi and blood and causing the development of abscesses. As the lungs and large intestine are interconnected, lung damage can also lead to the formation of abscesses in the large intestine.

Other potential causes include emotional disturbances, excessive hunger or fullness, strenuous physical labor, and carrying heavy loads. These factors may result in a disharmony between qi and blood, the generation of dampness and phlegm, and obstruction in the intestines, leading to the formation of abscesses. Initially, symptoms may include fever, aversion to cold, rapid and knotted pulse, changes in skin, hair, and nails, contraction of the right foot without extension, abdominal urgency progressing to swelling, and tenderness upon palpation, with a heavy sensation in the anus. Additionally, there may be difficulties in bowel movements, with the stool feeling heavy, and urinary symptoms such as hesitancy and a burning sensation.

Gu Shicheng, a physician from the Qing Dynasty, believed that the occurrence of sores, ulcers, and diarrhea could be attributed to several factors: it might be due to the damaging effect of cold and coolness, leading to a deficiency in spleen qi; or because of weak spleen qi, resulting in the inability to transform food; or due to spleen deficiency causing a downward sinking, unable to lift and hold; or because the gate of vitality fire is diminished, unable to generate earth (a metaphor for the spleen's function in Chinese medicine); or due to weakness in the kidney meridian, unable to contain; or because of spleen and kidney deficiency and cold, unable to perform their duties properly.

Chapter 8

Diagnosis and Treatment of Colon Cancer

Colon cancer, including both colon and rectal cancers, is a malignant disease caused by deficiencies in vital energy, internal damage due to diet, and emotional imbalances. It is characterized by the accumulation of damp-heat and toxic stasis in the intestines, leading to disrupted transmission within the digestive tract. The primary clinical manifestations include changes in bowel habits and stool characteristics, abdominal pain, anal prolapse pain, tenesmus, and even abdominal masses and weight loss. It is a common malignant tumor of the digestive tract. In North America and Western Europe, the incidence of colon cancer is still rising, ranking second among all cancer-related deaths. It mostly occurs in individuals aged 30-60 years, with a higher incidence in men than in women.

Etiology and Pathogenesis

THE DEVELOPMENT OF colon cancer is influenced by a combination of internal factors, such as deficiencies in vital energy, and external factors like the invasion of toxic pathogens. These factors interact with each other: deficiencies in vital energy make the body more susceptible to the invasion of toxic pathogens, further damaging the vital energy. When vital energy is weak and unable to resist pathogenic factors, these factors linger and accumulate in the large intestine. This accumulation leads to stagnation of qi (energy), blood, and toxins in the colon, causing obstruction and impaired transmission. Over time, these accumulations can develop into colon cancer.

1. Exogenous Damp-Heat: Residing in damp environments and being affected by external damp pathogenic factors can lead to dampness trapping the spleen, impairing its healthy functioning. This persistent internal and external dampness can provoke the disease.

2. Irregular Diet: Indulging in rich, greasy foods, alcoholic and fermented beverages, overeating cold or uncooked food, or binge eating and drinking can harm the spleen and stomach, leading to the generation of dampness. If this dampness is not dispelled and transforms into heat, it can descend to the large intestine, where it mixes with waste in the intestines. Over time, this can turn toxic, damaging the intestinal network and evolving into the disease.

3. Emotional Disturbances: Unfulfilled desires and frustrations can lead to stagnation of liver qi. Excessive liver wood attacking the spleen earth impairs the spleen's healthy functioning. This internal generation of dampness, which then stagnates and turns into heat, combines with damp-heat to affect the large intestine and can also trigger the disease.

4. Deficiency of Vital Energy: People with inherent deficiencies or those who are elderly and weak often have weakened spleen and kidney functions. The kidney is the foundation of congenital constitution, and the spleen is the basis of acquired constitution. Both organs are closely related to the transformation and transportation of dampness. The deficiency of these organs leads to internal retention of dampness, which over time can also lead to the disease.

The disease primarily affects the intestines but is closely related to the spleen, stomach, liver, and kidneys. In its early stages, the nature of the disease is mainly Damp-Heat and toxic stasis. In the late stages, it is characterized by deficiency of vital energy combined with the presence of pathogenic factors. The deficiency primarily involves spleen and kidney (qi) yang deficiency, deficiency of qi and blood, and liver and kidney yin deficiency. Exogenous damp-heat or damage to the spleen and stomach, leading to the internal generation of dampness that stagnates and turns into heat, is a significant cause of the disease. Long-term retention of damp-heat in the intestines, obstructing the flow of qi, and heat turning into poison, damaging the blood vessels, result in the accumulation of stagnated qi, damp-heat, toxins, and blood stasis in the intestines, forming masses, which is a key pathogenic mechanism of the disease.

Clinical Manifestations

THE BASIC CLINICAL manifestations of this disease include changes in bowel habits and stool characteristics, abdominal pain, a sensation of heaviness and pain in the anus, urgency followed by incomplete evacuation, and even the formation of abdominal masses.

1. Changes in Bowel Habits: This refers to an increase or decrease in the frequency of bowel movements, prolonged defecation time, etc. Changes in stool characteristics can manifest as frequent diarrhea, pasty or mucous stools, or constipation, with an alternation between diarrhea and constipation. There may also be blood in the stool or dysentery-like stools with pus and blood, and a change in the stool's shape, becoming flattened or thin.
2. Abdominal Pain: Often presents as continuous dull pain, but in cases of intestinal obstruction, the pain is typically colicky and accompanied by significant bloating.
3. Anal Heaviness and Urgency After Defecation: These symptoms often occur simultaneously and tend to worsen during defecation.
4. Abdominal Masses: Commonly found in the lower right abdomen, these masses are hard and fixed, with no tenderness

or only slight tenderness upon palpation.

Diagnosis

RECTAL DIGITAL EXAMINATION, total colonoscopy, barium enema X-ray examination, serum cancer embryonic antigen and colorectal cancer-related antigen testing, rectal ultrasound scanning, CT scans, and other examinations are used to confirm the diagnosis and assist in treatment.

Key Points for Syndrome Differentiation

The syndrome differentiation of this disease mainly involves distinguishing between rectal bleeding, stool shape, abdominal pain, and diarrhea to differentiate between deficiency and excess conditions.

1.Differentiating Rectal Bleeding: Rectal bleeding is a common symptom in patients with rectal cancer. The blood is often bright red, accompanied by a sensation of incomplete bowel movement and a burning sensation in the anus. This is caused by damp-heat descending and heat damaging the blood vessels.

2.Differentiating Stool Shape: Changes in stool to become thinner or flatter, often mixed with mucus or fresh blood, with progressively worsening symptoms, are due to the tumor continuously enlarging and obstructing the intestines.

3.Differentiating Abdominal Pain: Intermittent abdominal pain with no fixed location, which is somewhat relieved by defecation and passing gas, indicates Qi stagnation. Pain in a fixed location accompanied by an abdominal mass suggests blood stasis. Dull pain that is relieved by warmth indicates cold-deficiency; pain accompanied by spontaneous sweating or persistent dull pain indicates Qi and blood deficiency.

4. Differentiating Diarrhea: Irregular dry and loose stools are usually a sign of Qi stagnation. Diarrhea with pus and blood and a foul smell indicates damp-heat and toxic stasis. Chronic diarrhea or dysentery with

bowel sounds and temporary relief after defecation often points to cold-dampness. Thin, watery diarrhea followed by shortness of breath and dizziness after bowel movements suggests Qi and blood deficiency.

Treatment Principles

THE CENTRAL MECHANISM of this disease involves damp-heat, which further evolves into heat-toxin and stasis-toxin accumulating in the intestines, eventually forming masses over time. Therefore, the treatment principles are to clear heat, promote diuresis, dissipate stasis, and detoxify. In the late stages of the disease, when there is deficiency in healthy energy and excess in pathogenic factors, treatment should focus on nourishing deficiency while also detoxifying and dispersing masses, according to the different syndromes presented by the patient.

Differentiation on Diagnosis and Treatment

DAMP-HEAT SYNDROME

Symptoms: Abdominal colic, bloody or mucous stools, urgency and tenesmus, irregular bowel movements (either dry or loose), burning sensation in the anus, fever, nausea, chest stuffiness, dry mouth, yellow urine, red tongue with a greasy yellow coating, and a slippery and rapid pulse.

Treatment: Clear heat, promote dampness elimination, resolve stasis, and detoxify.

Stagnation of Blood and Toxins Syndrome

Symptoms: Abdominal resistance to pressure, or palpable masses in the abdomen, urgency and tenesmus, bloody and purulent stools, dark purple color with a large quantity, restlessness, heat sensation, thirst, dusky complexion, or the presence of ecchymosis and subcutaneous nodules. The tongue may appear dark purple with petechiae or ecchymosis, and the pulse is taut.

Treatment: Activate blood circulation, resolve stasis, clear heat, and detoxify.

Spleen and Kidney Yang Deficiency Syndrome

Symptoms: Abdominal pain relieved by warmth or pressure, or palpable masses in the abdomen, diarrhea with clear and watery stool or frequent bowel movements especially during the early morning, presence of blood in the stool, pale complexion, lack of energy, aversion to cold with cold limbs, soreness in the lower back and cold knees, thin white coating on the tongue, swollen and with toothmarks, and a deep, weak, and fine pulse.

Treatment: Warm and tonify the spleen and kidneys.

Qi and Blood Deficiency Syndrome

Symptoms: Persistent abdominal pain or palpable masses in the abdomen, sensation of heaviness or prolapse in the rectum, blood in the stool, diarrhea, pale complexion, lack of luster in the lips and nails, fatigue and weakness in the limbs, palpitations, shortness of breath, dizziness, thin body, poor appetite, thin white coating on the tongue, pale tongue, and a deep, fine, and weak pulse.

Treatment: Tonify Qi and nourish Blood.

Liver and Kidney Yin Deficiency Syndrome

Symptoms: Dull and lingering abdominal pain or palpable masses in the abdomen, constipation, blood in the stool, sore and weak lower back and knees, dizziness, tinnitus, blurred vision, sensation of heat in the chest, dryness in the mouth and throat, night sweats, spermatorrhea (involuntary discharge of semen), irregular menstruation, thin body, poor appetite, red tongue with little coating, and a wiry, thin, and rapid pulse.

Treatment: Nourish the kidneys and liver.

Please note that I have not listed the prescriptions of herbal formulas in this book as they should be applied by experienced TCM practitioners with proper training in TCM. Readers are advised to read my Chinese books for study and research purposes.

In the treatment of colorectal cancer, surgery, chemotherapy, and radiotherapy are definitely not the optimal options in the early and middle stages. Surgery easily leads to the metastasis of cancer cells, and there is a high possibility of causing symptoms in other organs. The focus should be on enhancing the patient's overall health and building a robust physique to resist the disease. Only in the advanced stages of colorectal cancer, when necessary, should methods like surgery be considered, and even then, caution should be exercised.

In the early stages of colorectal cancer, the predominant pattern is often damp-heat accumulation. However, as the disease progresses to the middle and late stages, especially after undergoing surgery, radiation, or chemotherapy, the clinical manifestations tend to transform towards a pattern characterized by spleen deficiency and blood depletion, indicating a shift from an excess condition to a deficiency condition.

If the medication is appropriately administered, and the body's vital energy is restored, the patient may have the potential for long-term survival.

Both patients and medical practitioners should note that the above method of differential diagnosis and treatment based on symptoms is a general approach found in modern TCM (Traditional Chinese Medicine) university textbooks on internal medicine, which is helpful for teaching and research. However, in actual clinical treatment, the conditions of patients can be more complicated, with some having combined syndromes or concurrent syndromes, and the conditions are constantly changing. Medical practitioners should not rigidly apply textbook dogmas, finding themselves at a loss, but should start from the comprehensive situation of the patient, analyze the specific conditions, make accurate diagnoses, differentiate and discuss treatment, and develop personalized treatment plans suitable for the actual situation of the patients. They should handle it calmly to achieve effectiveness.

Due to lifestyle and poor dietary habits being the main causes of colorectal cancer, there are many things that patients and their families can do. Assisting in improving the patient's lifestyle and dietary habits can contribute to enhancing their health, something that everyone can participate in and is not something that doctors can substitute. That's why I often say, everyone is their own best doctor. Therefore, the principles I discuss here are not just for medical professionals; patients and their families can and should listen, understand, and be aware. This way, the recovery of patients can be more efficient.